The Quick and Easy Collection for Beginners

Super-Affordable Seafood Recipes to Boost Your Metabolism and Eat Healthy

Naomi Hudson

Table of contents

Seafood-Stuffed Salmon Fillets

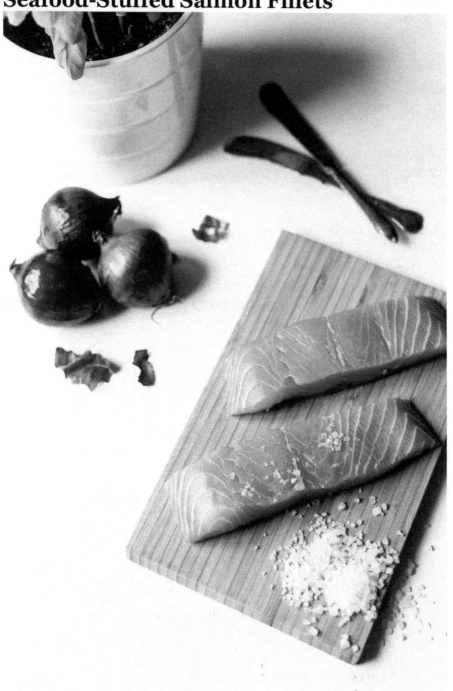

All out Time

Prep: 25 min. Heat: 20 min.

Makes

12 servings

Nutritional Facts

1 stuffed filet: 454 calories, 27g fat (6g immersed fat), 123mg cholesterol, 537mg sodium, 9g starch (0 sugars, 0 filaments), and 41g protein.

Ingredients

- 1-1/2 cups cooked long-grain rice

- 1 bundle (8 ounces) impersonation crabmeat

- 2 tablespoons cream cheddar, relaxed

- 2 tablespoons margarine, dissolved

- 2 garlic cloves, minced

- 1/2 teaspoon each dried basil, marjoram, oregano, thyme, and rosemary, squashed

- 1/2 teaspoon celery seed, squashed

- 12 salmon filets (8 ounces each and 1-1/2 inches thick)

- 3 tablespoons olive oil

- 2 teaspoons dill weed

- 1-1/2 teaspoons salt

Direction

1.   Preheat stove to 400°. In an enormous bowl, join rice, crab, cream cheddar, spread, garlic, basil, marjoram, oregano, thyme, rosemary,

and celery seed.

2.   Cut a pocket on a level plane in each filet to inside 1/2 in. of the inverse side. Load up with stuffing blend; secure with

toothpicks. Spot salmon on 2 lubed 15x10x1-in. heating skillet. Brush with oil; sprinkle with dill and salt.

3.   Bake 18-22 minutes or until fish just starts to chip effectively with a fork. Dispose of toothpicks before serving.

Classic Crab Boil

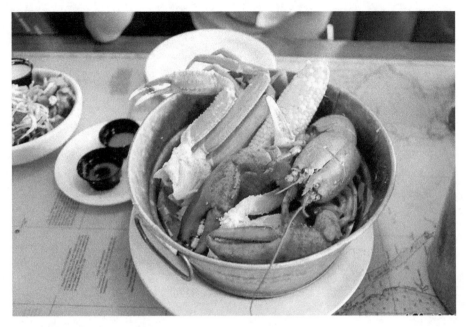

All out Time

Prep: 10 min. Cook: 30 min.

Makes

2 servings

Nutritional Facts

1 crab: 245 calories, 3g fat (0 immersed fats), 169mg cholesterol, 956mg sodium, 2g starch (0 sugars, 0 fiber), 50g protein.

Ingredients

- 2 tablespoons mustard seed

- 2 tablespoons celery seed

- 1 tablespoon dill seed

- 1 tablespoon coriander seeds

- 1 tablespoon entire allspice

- ½ teaspoon entire cloves

- 4 cove leaves

- Cheesecloth

- 8 quarts water

- ¼ cup salt

- ¼ cup lemon juice

- 1 teaspoon cayenne pepper

- 2 entire live Dungeness crab (2 pounds each)

Melted margarine and lemon wedges Directions

1.   Place the initial seven fixings on a twofold thickness of cheesecloth. Assemble corners of fabric to encase seasonings; tie safely with string.

2.   In an enormous stockpot, bring water, salt, lemon juice, cayenne and flavor sack to a bubble. Utilizing tongs add crab to stockpot; come back to a bubble. Decrease heat; stew, secured, until shells turn splendid red, around 15 minutes.

3.   Using tongs, expel crab from the pot. Dash under virus water or dive into ice water. Present with dissolved margarine and lemon wedges.

Foil-Packet Shrimp and Sausage Jambalaya

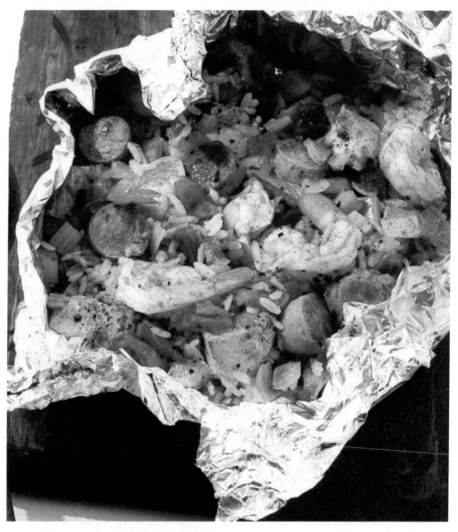

All out Time

Prep: 20 min. Heat: 20 min.

Makes

6 servings

1 parcel: 287 calories, 12g fat (4g immersed fat), 143mg cholesterol, 1068mg sodium, 23g starch (3g sugars, 2g fiber), 23g protein.

Ingredients

- 12 ounces completely cooked andouille wiener joins, cut into 1/2-inch cuts

- 12 ounces uncooked shrimp (31-40 for every pound), stripped and deveined

- 1 medium green pepper, slashed
-
- 1 medium onion, slashed

- 2 celery ribs, slashed

- 3 garlic cloves, minced

- 2 teaspoons Creole flavoring

- 1 can (14-1/2 ounces) fire-simmered diced tomatoes, depleted

- 1 cup uncooked moment rice

- 1 can (8 ounces) tomato sauce

- 1/2 cup chicken juices

Directions

1.   Preheat broiler to 425°. In an enormous bowl, join all fixings. Partition blend among 6 lubed 18x12-in. Bits of substantial foil. Crease foil around blend and pleat edges to seal, framing bundles; place on a heating sheet. Prepare until shrimp turn pink and rice is delicate, 20-25 minutes.

Lemony Scallops with Angel Hair Pasta

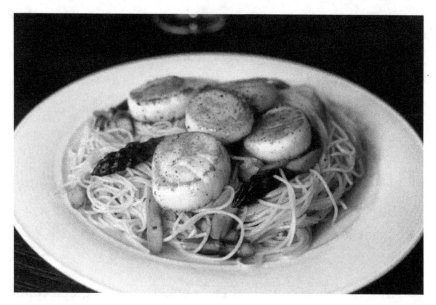

Complete Time

Prep/Total Time: 25 min.

Makes

4   servings Nourishment Facts

1-1/2 cups: 404 calories, 13g fat (2g soaked fat), 27mg cholesterol, 737mg sodium, 48g starch (4g sugars, 6g fiber), and 25g protein.

Ingredients

8 ounces uncooked multigrain holy messenger hair pasta

- 3 tablespoons olive oil, separated

- 1 pound ocean scallops, tapped dry

- 2 cups cut radishes (around 1 pack)

- 2 garlic cloves, cut

- 1/2 teaspoon squashed red pepper chips 6 green onions, daintily cut 1/2 teaspoon legitimate salt

- 1 tablespoon ground lemon get-up-and-go 1/4 cup lemon juice

Directions

2.   In a 6-qt. stockpot, cook pasta as per bundle bearings; channel and come back to the pot.

3.   Meanwhile, in a huge skillet, heat 2 tablespoons oil over medium-high warmth; singe scallops in clusters until misty and

edges are brilliant darker, around 2 minutes for every side. Expel from skillet; keep warm.

4.   In a similar skillet, saute radishes, garlic and pepper chips in residual oil until radishes are delicate, 2-3 minutes. Mix in green onions and salt; cook 1 moment. Add to pasta; hurl to consolidate. Sprinkle with lemon pizzazz and juice. Top with scallops to serve.

Pan-Seared Salmon with Dill Sauce

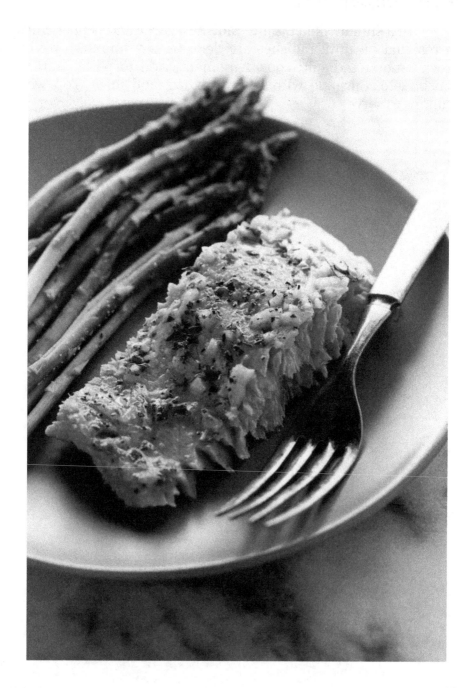

Complete Time

Prep/Total Time: 25 min.

Makes

4 servings

Nourishment Facts

1 salmon filet with 1/4 cup sauce: 366 calories, 25g fat (4g soaked fat), 92mg cholesterol, 349mg sodium, 4g starch (3g sugars, 0 fibers), 31g protein. Diabetic trades: 4 lean meat, 2-1/2 fat.

Ingredients:

- 1 tablespoon canola oil

- 4 salmon filets (6 ounces each)

- 1 teaspoon Italian flavoring

- 1/4 teaspoon salt

- 1/2 cup decreased fat plain yogurt

- 1/4 cup decreased fat mayonnaise

- 1/4 cup finely hacked cucumber

- 1 teaspoon cut crisp dill

Directions

1.   In a huge skillet, heat oil over medium-high warmth. Sprinkle salmon with Italian flavoring and salt. A spot in skillet, skin side down. Lessen warmth to medium. Cook until fish just starts to drop effectively with a fork, around 5 minutes on each side.

2.   Meanwhile, in a little bowl, join yogurt, mayonnaise, cucumber, and dill. Present with salmon.

Broiled Tilapia

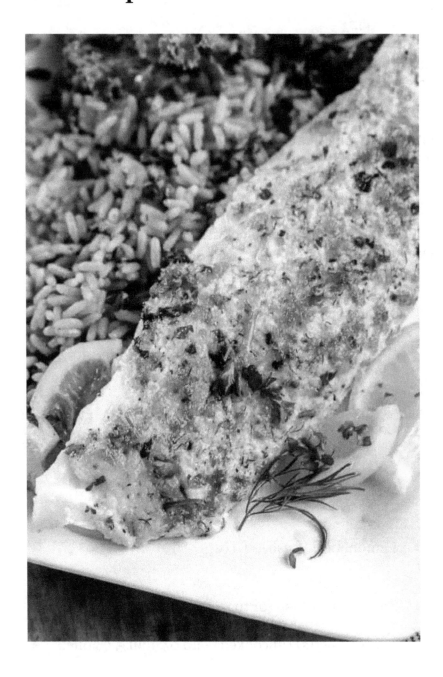

SmartPoints value: Green plan - 2SP, Blue plan - 0SP, Purple plan - 0SP

Total Time: 13 min, Prep time: 8 min, Cooking time: 5 min, Serves: 4

Nutritional value: Cal - 154.8, Carbs - 1.5g, Fat - 6.4g, Protein - 22.8g

You can apply this recipe with other types of fish, such as sole, halibut, flounder, and even shellfish. You also swap lime juice for lemon juice.

Ingredients

- Black pepper - ¼ tsp, freshly ground

- Cooking spray - 1 spray(s)

- Garlic (herb seasoning) - 2 tsp

- Lemon juice (fresh) - 1 Tbsp

- Table salt - ½ tsp (or to taste)

- Tilapia fillet(s) (uncooked) - 20 oz, four 5 oz fillets

Instructions

1.   Prepare your grill by preheating. Coat a skillet with cooking spray.

2.   Apply seasoning to both sides of the fish with salt and pepper.

3.   Transfer the fish to the prepared skillet and drizzle it with lemon juice, then sprinkle garlic herb seasoning over the top.

4.   Broil the fish until it is fork-tender; about 5 minutes.

Grilled Miso-Glazed Cod

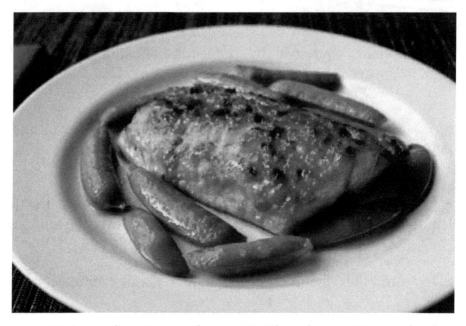

SmartPoints value: Green plan - 3SP, Blue plan - 2SP, Purple plan - 2SP

Total Time: 35 min, Prep time: 10 min, Cooking time: 15 min, Serves: 4

Nutritional value: Cal - 227.2, Carbs - 15.0g, Fat - 3.1g, Protein - 30.0g

This marinade produces a fantastic glaze for grilled cod. You can pair it with grilled scallions, drizzled with low-sodium soy sauce, and sesame oil to make a complete meal. If you don't have a fish basket, put foil on one area of your grill to prevent the fish from sticking out below it. Alternatively, you can broil the fish instead. Cod makes a perfect choice for grilling. Flip the fish when it starts to flake and turn opaque. Use a spatula with a broader mouth when turning the fish to help prevent the fish from breaking apart when turning. It is preferable to serve this dish with roasted carrots or broccoli.

Ingredients

- White miso - 3 Tbsp

- Sugar (dark brown) - 1½ Tbsp

- Sake - 1 Tbsp

- Mirin - ½ fl oz, (1 Tbsp)

- Atlantic cod (uncooked) - 20 oz, (fillets, skin removed

- Cooking spray - 1 spray(s)

- Uncooked scallion(s) (chopped) - 2 Tbsp

Instructions

1.   Whisk together miso, sugar, sake, and mirin in a small bowl and spread the mixture over the cod. Cover the cod and refrigerate for at least 2 hours or up to 24 hours.

2.   Coat a grill pan off the heat with cooking spray and preheat to medium heat.

3.   Remove the cod from marinade (reserve marinade). Place it in a fish grilling basket and grill until the cod is opaque and flakes easily with a fork.

4.   Grill each side for about 5 to 7 min (brush the cod with the remaining marinade half-way through the grilling phase to create a thicker glaze). Serve the cod garnished with scallions.

Grilled Tuna with Herb Butter

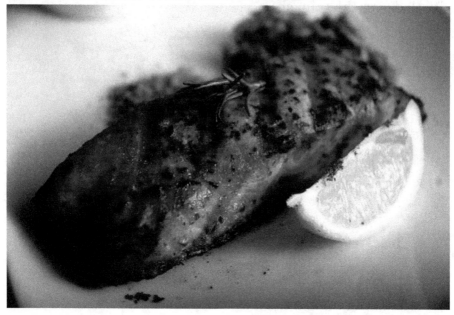

SmartPoints value: Green plan - 4SP, Blue plan - 3SP, Purple plan - 3SP

Total Time: 18 min, Prep time: 12 min, Cooking time: 6 min, Serves: 4

Nutritional value: Calories - 192.0, Carbs - 8.3g, Fat - 2.5g, Protein - 38.3g

You can prepare this grilled tuna recipe in under 20 minutes. Drizzle some olive oil and lime over the tuna before you start cooking it for a unique flavor. You can nicely substitute with a lemon if you don't have a lime. I will recommend that you use salted butter for the sauce instead of unsalted butter to enhance the flavor of the dish. The secret ingredient in this grilled fish recipe is the freshly made herb butter. It also tastes great when drizzled over the spinach.

Ingredients

- Olive oil - 1 tsp

- Lime juice (fresh) - 1 tsp

- Black pepper - ⅛ tsp, or to taste

- Cooking spray - 1 spray(s)

- Salted butter - 2 Tbsp, softened

- Chives (finely chopped) - 1 Tbsp, fresh

- Parsley (fresh) - 1 Tbsp, finely chopped

- Tarragon (fresh) - 1 Tbsp, finely chopped

- Lime zest (fresh, minced) - 1 tsp

- Table salt - ¼ tsp, or to taste

- Spinach (fresh) - 1 pound(s), baby-variety, steamed

- Yellowfin tuna (uncooked) - 1 pound(s), one steak cut 1- to 1-1/2 inches thick

Instructions

1.   Drizzle oil and lime juice on both sides of the fish and set it aside.

2.   Coat your grill with cooking spray off heat, and preheat the grill on high heat.

3.   Combine softened butter, chives, parsley, tarragon, lime zest, salt, and pepper in a small metal bowl and then set aside.

4.   Grill the tuna on one side for three minutes, then carefully turn it and cook on the other side for another three minutes or longer until you have achieved the desired degree of cooking.

5.   Place the bowl containing butter mixture on the grill just until it melts. Don't let it cook.

6.   Slice the tuna thinly and serve it over spinach, then drizzle melted herb butter over the top.

Notes: If you prefer, you can broil the tuna on a grill pan. In this recipe, you will prepare the tuna like a steak. In case you prefer your tuna to be more well done, add about 1 minute to your total cooking time. However, tuna cooks rapidly, so make sure you do not overcook it. The herb butter is excellent on both the tuna and the spinach.

Lemon-Herb Roasted Salmon

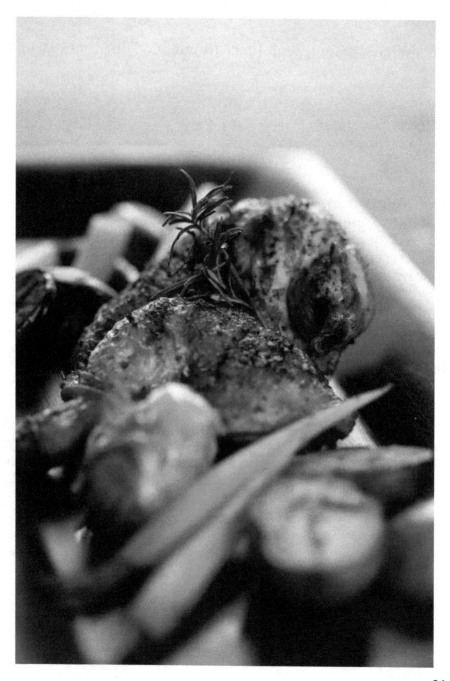

SmartPoints value: Green plan - 5SP, Blue plan - 2SP, Purple plan - 2SP

Total Time: 31 min, Prep time: 16 min, Cooking time: 15 min, Serves: 4

Nutritional value: Calories - 118.1, Carbs - 1.0g, Fat - 6.8g, Protein - 12.9g

Give your family a fabulous salmon flavor with lemon juice, lemon zest, and fresh herbs in this easy entrée that will be ready in about 30 minutes. I have used pink salmon fillets because they are less fatty compared to some other salmon varieties like sockeye and Coho salmon.

The salmon should flake when pierced with a fork. That's an excellent indicator that it is ready. Ensure that you zest the lemon before juicing it.

To produce enough zest and juice for this recipe, you will need about two lemons. The mix of fresh herbs in this dish is lovely. However, you can use whatever combination you like; this recipe is versatile. Stir a few red pepper flakes into the herb mixture to add a little heat.

Ingredients

- Black pepper (coarsely ground) - ⅛ tsp (or to taste)

- Cooking spray - 1 spray(s)

- Lemon juice (fresh) - 4 Tbsp, divided

- Lemon zest (finely grated) - 1 tsp (with extra for garnish, if you like)

- Minced garlic - 1 tsp

- Oregano (fresh) - 1 tsp

- Parsley (fresh, chopped) - 1 Tbsp (with extra for garnish, if you like)

- Uncooked wild pink salmon fillet(s) (also known as humpback salmon) - 1½ pound(s), four 6-oz pieces about 1-inch-thick each

- Table salt - ⅛ tsp (or to taste)

- Sugar - 1½ Tbsp

- Thyme (fresh, chopped) - 1 Tbsp (with extra for garnish, if you like)

Instructions

1.   Heat your oven to 400°F before using it. Get a small, shallow baking dish and coat it with cooking spray.

2.   Apply seasoning to both sides of the salmon with salt and pepper, then place the salmon in the prepared baking dish and drizzle on it with two tablespoons of lemon juice.

3.   Whisk the remaining two tablespoons of lemon juice, sugar, parsley, thyme, lemon zest, garlic, and oregano together in a small bowl, then continue whisking until the sugar dissolves in the mixture and set it aside.

4.   Roast the salmon until it is close to being ready; about 13 minutes, then remove it from the oven and top it with the lemon-herb mixture.

5.   Return it to the oven and allow it to roast until the salmon is fork-tender, about 2 minutes more. Garnish the dish with fresh herbs that you chopped and the grated zest, if you like.

Grilled Tuna Provencal

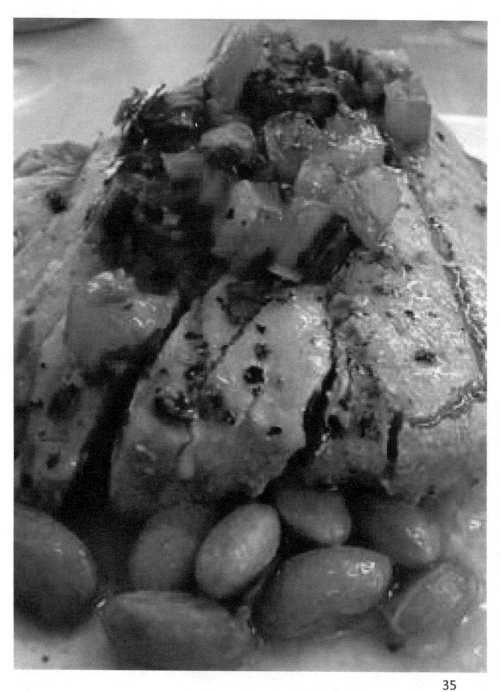

SmartPoints value: Green plan - 3SP, Blue plan - 2SP, Purple plan - 2SP

Total Time: 20 min, Prep time: 10 min, Cooking time: 10 min, Serves: 4

Nutritional value: Calories - 335, Carbs - 14.6g, Fat - 15.5g, Protein - 36.1g

This one-dish meal is usually ready in just 20 minutes, oozing with a delicious French flavor. You can make the whole meal in one pan, aiding clean up after cooking. To cook with a grill pan and get the best result, you need to preheat the pan for at least five minutes to ensure that you distribute the heat evenly. That will help you avoid overcooking parts of the meat while not cooking other parts. If you're not sure about the hotness of the grill pan, drop a half teaspoon of water on there to see if it evaporates.

With steamed spinach or a bed of rice, this dish tastes lovely.

Ingredients

- Black pepper (freshly ground, divided) - ¾ tsp

- Cooking spray - 3 spray(s)

- Uncooked tuna (about 1- to 1 1/2-in thick) - 1 pound(s)

- Olive(s) (pitted and chopped)- 6 large

- Olive oil - 1 Tbsp

- Rosemary (fresh, minced) - 1 Tbsp

- Red wine - 2 fl oz

- Sea salt - ¾ tsp, divided

- Tomato(es) (fresh, diced) - 2½ cup(s)

- Garlic clove(s) (minced) - 2 medium clove(s)

- Parsley (fresh, minced) - 2 Tbsp

- Sugar - ⅛ tsp

Instructions

1.   Wash the tuna thoroughly and pat it dry. Rub 1/4 teaspoon each of salt and pepper over it, then set it aside.

2.   Combine tomatoes, parsley, rosemary, garlic, olives, oil, and the remaining 1/2 teaspoon each of salt and pepper in a separate bowl,

then set it aside.

3.   Get a reasonably large grill pan and coat it with cooking spray, then set it over medium-high heat. When the pan is visibly hot, cook the tuna for 2 to 3 minutes (or longer) per side for a rare cook (or thorough cook). As soon as you have prepared the tuna, remove it to a serving plate and wrap it with aluminum foil to keep it warm.

4.   Add the red wine, tomato mixture, and sugar to the hot grill pan and cook, scraping the bottom of the pan frequently, until the tomato mixture reduces to about two cups. The alcohol must have cooked off.

5.   Remove foil from the tuna, slice it thinly, and serve with tomato mixture over the top.

Grilled Cod Fillets with Lemon Dill Butter

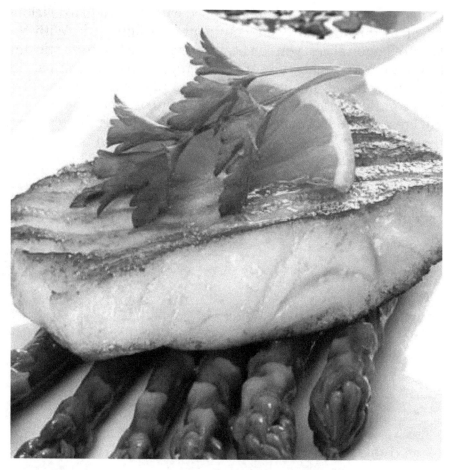

SmartPoints value: Green plan - 3SP, Blue plan - 2SP, Purple plan - 2SP

Total Time: 25 min, Prep time: 15 min, Cooking time: 10 min, Serves: 4

Nutritional value: Calories - 318.7g, Carbs - 6.7g, Fat - 13.0g, Protein - 41.7g

Grill the fish on slices of lemon topped with dill to add a delicious flavor to this dish. Become confident at grilling fish. With the layer of lemon slices, you can easily prevent the fish from sticking to the grate. To make use of a stovetop, prepare a grill pan by preheating it over medium-high heat until it is almost smoking, then continue with the recipe. The mixture of lemon, butter, and dill creates a robust sauce that becomes ready in minutes, even though it tastes like you spent hours preparing it. It is preferable to serve this dish with grilled asparagus.

Ingredients

- Olive oil -2 tsp

- Uncooked Atlantic cod - 24 oz, or another firm white fish like

- tilapia (four 6-oz fillets)

- Table salt - ½ tsp

- Lemon(s) (sliced 1/4-in thick) - 2 medium (you'll need 12 slices total)

- Dill - 2 tsp, chopped

- Dill - 4 sprig(s)

- Light butter - 4 tsp (at room temp.)

- Lemon zest - 1 tsp

Instructions

1.   Get your grill ready by preheating to medium-high heat. Continue the heating for at least 10 minutes after it reaches the desired temperature, then scrape the grate clean with a steel brush and coat it lightly with oil.

2.   While the grill heats up, pat the fish dry and sprinkle salt on it.

3.   Place three lemon slices on the grill carefully, overlapping slightly, and top it with a dill sprig and fish fillet.

4.   Repeat the same with the remaining lemon, dill, and fish. Cover the grill and cook without turning for 8-10 minutes until the fish is opaque all the way through and yields easily to a thin-bladed knife.

5.   While the cooking is on-going, mix the butter, chopped dill, and zest in a small shallow bowl.

6.   Transfer each lemon-dill-fish portion to a plate using two thin-bladed spatulas and top them with 1 1/2 tsp of lemon-dill butter and serve (serving the lemon slices is optional).

Spicy Baked Shrimp

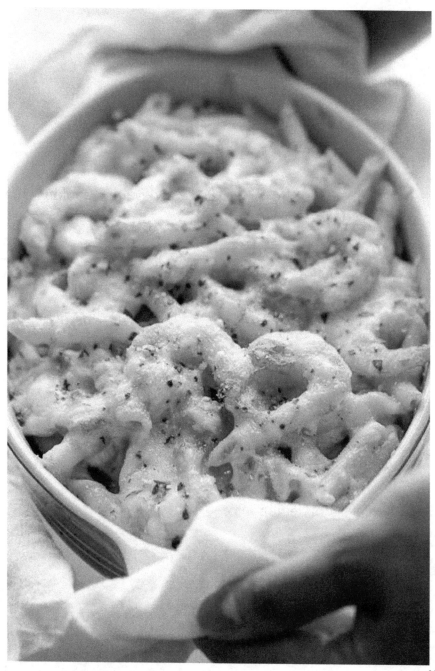

Serving: 4

Prep Time: 10 minutes

Cook Time: 25 minutes + 2-4 hours

Ingredients:

- ½ ounce large shrimp, peeled and deveined Cooking spray as needed

- 1 teaspoon low sodium coconut amines

- 1 teaspoon parsley

- ½ teaspoon olive oil

- ½ tablespoon honey

- 1 tablespoon lemon juice

How To:

1.	Pre-heat your oven to 450 degrees F.

2.   Take a baking dish and grease it well.

3.   Mix altogether the ingredients and toss.

4.   Transfer to oven and bake for 8 minutes until shrimp turns pink.

5.   Serve and enjoy!

Nutrition (Per Serving)

Calories: 321

Fat: 9g

Carbohydrates: 44g

Protein: 22g

Shrimp and Cilantro Meal

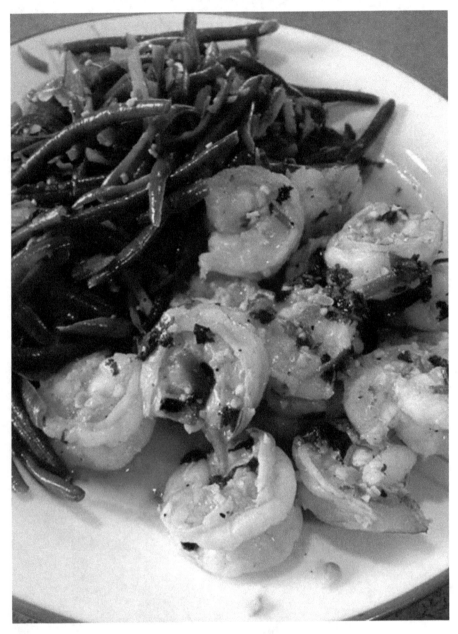

Serving: 4

Prep Time: 10 minutes

Cook Time: 5 minutes

Ingredients:

- ¾ pounds shrimp, deveined and peeled

- tablespoons fresh lime juice

- ¼ teaspoon cloves, minced

- ½ teaspoon ground cumin

- 1 tablespoon olive oil

- 1 ¼ cups fresh cilantro, chopped

- 1 teaspoon lime zest

- ½ teaspoon sunflower seeds
- ¼ teaspoon pepper

Direction

1.   Take an outsized sized bowl and add shrimp, cumin, garlic, juice , ginger and toss well.

2.   Take an outsized sized non-stick skillet and add oil, allow the oil to

heat up over medium-high heat.

3.   Add shrimp mixture and sauté for 4 minutes.

4.   Remove the warmth and add cilantro, lime zest, sunflower seeds, and pepper.

5.   Mix well and serve hot!

Nutrition (Per Serving)

Calories: 177

Fat: 6g

Carbohydrates: 2g

Protein: 27g

The Original Dijon Fish

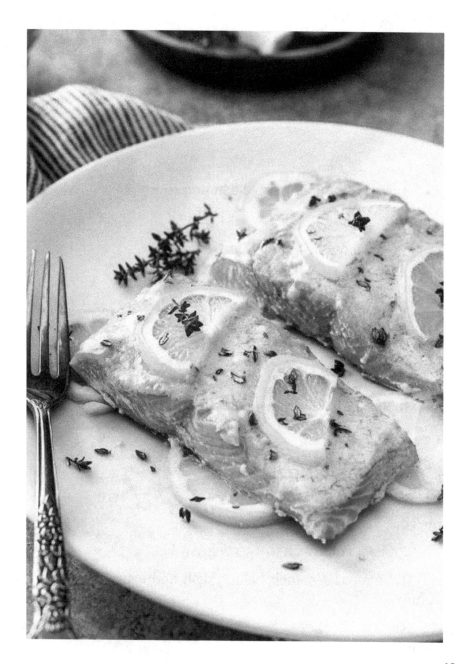

Serving: 2

Prep Time: 3 minutes

Cook Time: 12 minutes

Ingredients:

- 1 perch, flounder or sole fish florets

- 1 tablespoon Dijon mustard

- 1 ½ teaspoons lemon juice

- teaspoon low sodium Worcestershire sauce, low sodium

- tablespoons Italian seasoned bread crumbs

- 1 almond butter flavored cooking spray

How To:

1.   Preheat your oven to 450 degrees F.

2.   Take an 11 x 7-inch baking dish and arrange your fillets carefully.

3.   Take a little sized bowl and add juice, Worcester sauce, mustard and blend it well.

4.   Pour the combination over your fillet.

5.   Sprinkle an honest amount of breadcrumbs.

6.   Bake for 12 minutes until fish flakes off easily.

7.   Cut the fillet in half portions and enjoy!

Nutrition (Per Serving)

Calories: 125

Fat: 2g

Carbohydrates: 6g

Protein: 21g

Lemony Garlic Shrimp

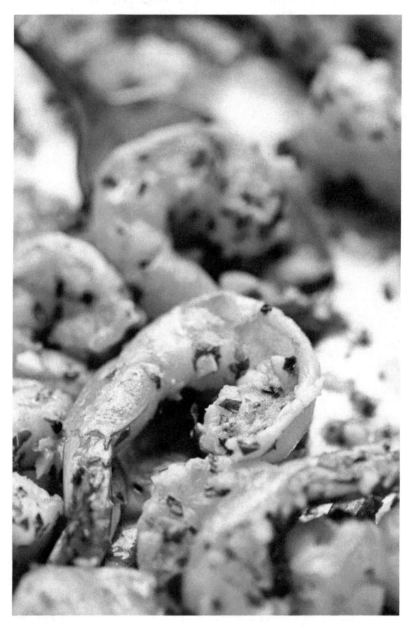

Serving: 4

Prep Time: 5-10 minutes

Cook Time: 10-15 minutes

Ingredients:

- 1 ¼ pounds shrimp, boiled or steamed

- tablespoons garlic, minced

- ¼ cup lemon juice

- tablespoons olive oil

- ¼ cup parsley

How To:

1.　Take alittle skillet and place over medium heat, add garlic and oil and stir-cook for 1 minute.

2.　Add parsley, juice and season with sunflower seeds and pepper accordingly.

3.   Add shrimp during a large bowl and transfer the mixture from the skillet over the shrimp.

4.   Chill and serve.

5.   Enjoy!

Nutrition (Per Serving)

Calories: 130

Fat: 3g

Carbohydrates:2g

Protein:22g

Baked Zucchini Wrapped Fish

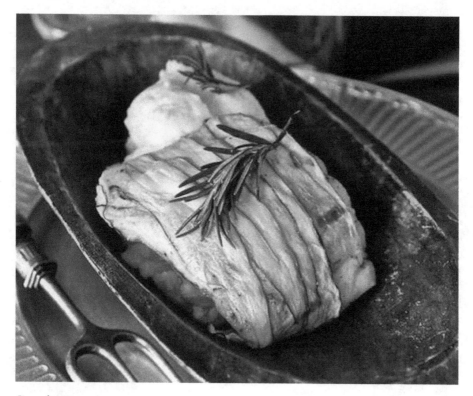

Serving: 2

Prep Time: 15 minutes

Cook Time: 15 minutes

Ingredients:

- 24-ounce cod fillets, skin removed

- tablespoon of blackening spices

- zucchini, sliced lengthwise to form ribbon

- ½ tablespoon of olive oil

How To:

1. Season the fish fillets with blackening spice.

2. Wrap each fillet with zucchini ribbons.
3. Place fish on a plate.
4. Take a skillet and place over medium heat.
5. Pour oil and permit the oil to heat up.
6. Add wrapped fish to the skillet and cook all sides for 4 minutes.

7. Serve and enjoy!

Nutrition (Per Serving)

Calories: 397

Fat: 23g

Carbohydrates: 2g

Protein: 46g

Heart-Warming Medi Tilapia

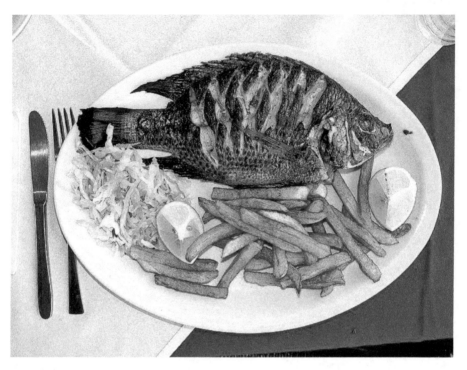

Serving: 4

Prep Time: 15 minutes

Cook Time: 15 minute

Ingredients:

- tablespoons sun-dried tomatoes, packed in oil, drained and

- chopped

- tablespoon capers, drained

- tilapia fillets

- tablespoon oil from sun-dried tomatoes

- tablespoons kalamata olives, chopped and pitted

How To:

1. Pre-heat your oven to 372 degrees F.

2. Take alittle sized bowl and add sun-dried tomatoes, olives, capers and stir well.

3. Keep the mixture on the side.

4. Take a baking sheet and transfer the tilapia fillets and arrange them side by side.

5. Drizzle vegetable oil everywhere them.

6. Bake in your oven for 10-15 minutes.

7. After 10 minutes, check the fish for a "Flaky" texture.

8. Once cooked, top the fish with the tomato mixture and serve!

Nutrition (Per Serving)

Calories: 183

Fat: 8g

Carbohydrates: 18g

Protein:83g

Baked Salmon and Orange Juice

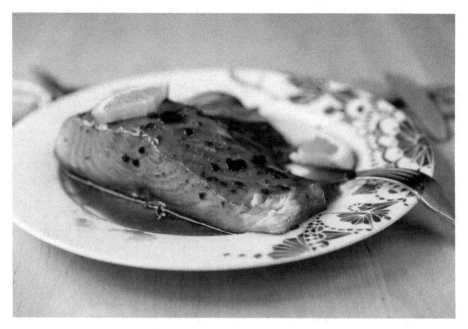

Serving: 2

Prep Time: 10 minutes

Cook Time: 10 minutes

Ingredients:

- ½ pound salmon steak

- Juice of 1 orange

- Pinch ginger powder, black pepper, and sunflower seeds

- Juice of ½ lemon

- 1-ounce coconut almond milk

How To:

1. Preheat oven to 350 degrees F.
2. Rub salmon steak with spices and let it sit for quarter-hour.
3. Take a bowl and squeeze an orange.
4. Squeeze juice also and blend .
5. Pour almond milk into the mixture and stir.
6. Take a baking dish and line with aluminium foil .
7. Place steak thereon and pour the sauce over steak.
8. Cover with another sheet and bake for 10 minutes.
9. Serve and enjoy!

Nutrition (Per Serving)

Calories: 300

Fat: 3g

Carbohydrates: 1g

Protein: 7g

Lemon and Almond butter Cod

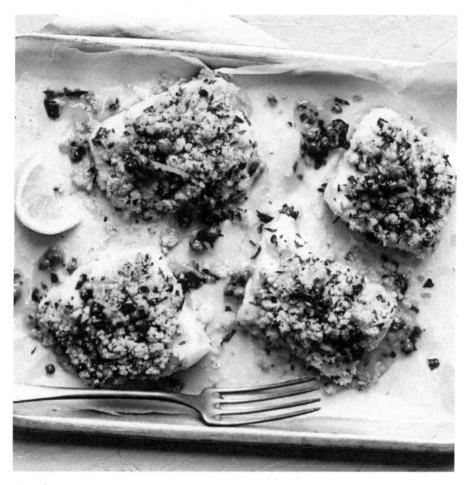

Serving: 2

Prep Time: 5 minutes

Cook Time: 20 minutes

Ingredients:

- tablespoons almond butter, divided thyme sprigs, fresh and divided

- 5 teaspoons lemon juice, fresh and divided

- cod fillets, 6 ounces each Sunflower seeds to taste

How To:

1.   Pre-heat your oven to 400 degrees F.

2.   Season cod fillets with sunflower seeds on each side .

3.   Take four pieces of foil, each foil should be 3 times bigger than the fillets.

4.   Divide fillets between the foil and top with almond butter, juice ,thyme.

5.   Fold to make a pouch and transfer pouches to the baking sheet.

6.   Bake for 20 minutes.

7.   Open and let the steam out.

8.   Serve and enjoy!

Nutrition (Per Serving)

Calories: 284

Fat: 18g

Carbohydrates: 2g

Protein: 32g

Shrimp Scampi

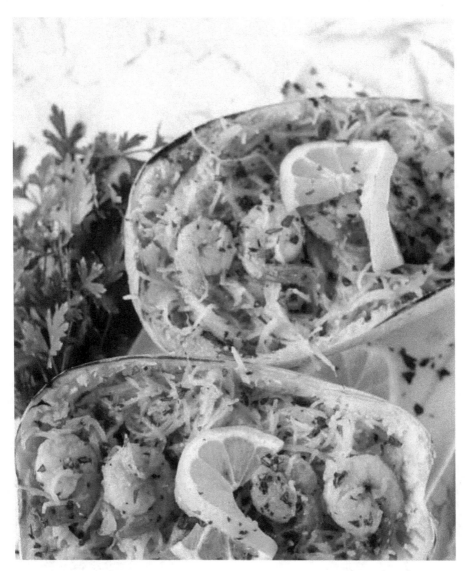

Serving: 4

Prep Time: 25 minutes

Cook Time: Nil

Ingredients:

- teaspoons olive oil

- 1 ¼ pounds medium shrimp

- 6-8 garlic cloves, minced

- ½ cup low sodium chicken broth

- ½ cup dry white wine

- ¼ cup fresh lemon juice

- ¼ cup fresh parsley + 1 tablespoon extra, minced

- ¼ teaspoon sunflower seeds

- ¼ teaspoon fresh ground pepper

- slices lemon

How To:

1.　　Take an outsized sized bowl and place it over medium-high heat.

2.　　Add oil and permit the oil to heat up.

3.　　Add shrimp and cook for 2-3 minutes.

4.　　Add garlic and cook for 30 seconds.

5.　　Take a slotted spoon and transfer the cooked shrimp to a serving platter.

6.　　Add broth, juice , wine, ¼ cup of parsley, pepper, and sunflower seeds to the skillet.

7.　　Bring the entire mix to a boil.

8.　　Keep boiling until the sauce has been reduced to half.

9.　　Spoon the sauce over the cooked shrimp.

10.　　Garnish with parsley and lemon.

11.　　Serve and enjoy!

Nutrition (Per Serving)

Calories: 184

Fat: 6g

Carbohydrates: 6g

Protein: 15g

Lemon and Garlic Scallops

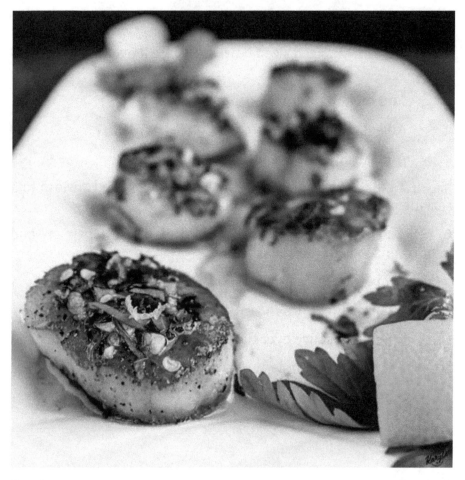

Serving: 4

Prep Time: 10 minutes

Cook Time: 5 minutes

Ingredients:

- 1 tablespoon olive oil

- ¼ pounds dried scallops

- tablespoons all-purpose flour

- ¼ teaspoon sunflower seeds

- 4-5 garlic cloves, minced

- 1 scallion, chopped

- 1 pinch of ground sage

- lemon juice

- tablespoons parsley, chopped

Direction

1.   Take a non-stick skillet and place over medium-high heat.

2.   Add oil and permit the oil to heat up.

3.   Take a medium sized bowl and add scallops alongside sunflower seeds and flour.

4.   Place the scallops within the skillet and add scallions, garlic, and sage.

5.   Sauté for 3-4 minutes until they show an opaque texture.

6.   Stir in juice and parsley.

7.   Remove heat and serve hot!

Nutrition (Per Serving)

Calories: 151

Fat: 4g

Carbohydrates: 10g

Protein: 18g

Walnut Encrusted Salmon

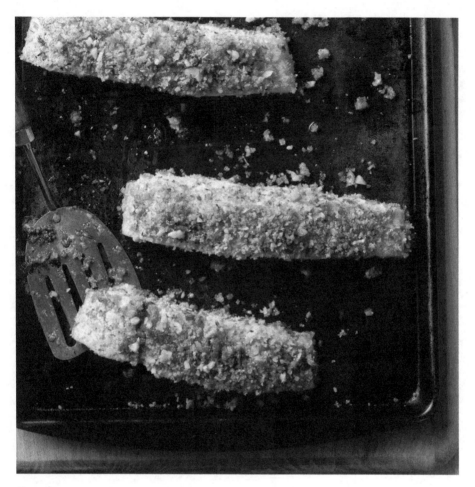

Serving: 34

Prep Time: 10 minutes

Cook Time: 14 minutes

Ingredients:

- ½ cup walnuts

- tablespoons stevia

- ½ tablespoon Dijon mustard

- ¼ teaspoon dill

- salmon fillets (3 ounces each)

- 1 tablespoon olive oil

- Sunflower seeds and pepper to taste

How To:

1.   Pre-heat your oven to 350 degrees F.

2.   Add walnuts, mustard, stevia to kitchen appliance and process until your required consistency is achieved.

3.   Take a frypan and place it over medium heat.

4.   Add oil and let it heat up.

5. Add salmon and sear for 3 minutes.

6. Add walnut mix and coat well.

7. Transfer coated salmon to baking sheet, bake in oven for 8 minutes.

8. Serve and enjoy!

Nutrition (Per Serving)

Calories: 373

Fat: 43g

Carbohydrates: 4g

Protein: 20g

Roasted Lemon Swordfish

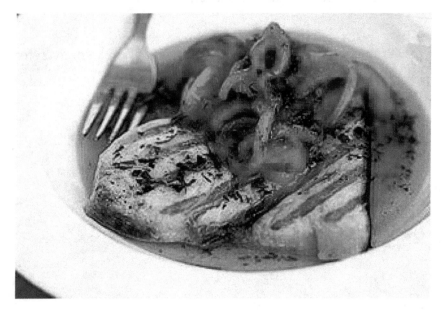

Serving: 4

Prep Time: 10 minutes

Cook Time: 70-80 minutes

Ingredients:

- ¼ cup parsley, chopped

- ½ teaspoon garlic, chopped

- ½ teaspoon canola oil

- swordfish fillets, 6 ounces each

- ¼ teaspoon sunflower seeds

- tablespoon sugar

- lemons, quartered and seeds removed

How To:

1.   Preheat your oven to 375 degrees F.

2.   Take a small-sized bowl and add sugar, sunflower seeds, lemon wedges.

3.   Toss well to coat them.

4.   Take a shallow baking dish and add lemons, cover with aluminum foil .

5.   Roast for about hour until lemons are tender and browned (Slightly).

6.   Heat your grill and place the rack about 4 inches far away from the source of warmth .

7.   Take a baking pan and coat it with cooking spray.

8.   Transfer fish fillets to the pan and brush with oil on top spread garlic on top.

9.   Grill for about 5 minutes all sides until fillet turns opaque.

10.   Transfer fish to a serving platter, squeeze roasted

lemon on top.

11.   Sprinkle parsley, serve with a lemon wedge on the

side.

12.   Enjoy!

Nutrition (Per Serving)

Calories: 280

Fat: 12g

Net Carbohydrates: 4g

Protein: 34g

Especial Glazed Salmon

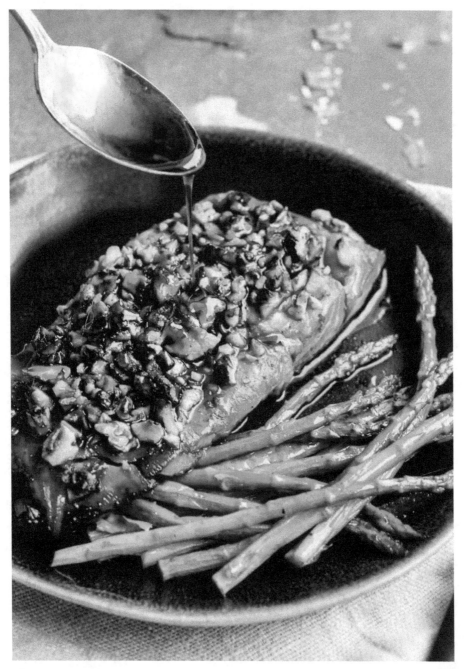

Serving: 4

Prep Time: 45 minutes

Cook Time: 10 minutes

Ingredients:

- Pieces of salmon fillets, 5 ounces each

- tablespoons coconut aminos

- Teaspoon olive oil

- 2 teaspoons ginger, minced

- teaspoons garlic, minced

- 2 tablespoons sugar-free ketchup

- tablespoons dry white wine

- 2 tablespoons red boat fish sauce, low sodium

How To:

1.   Take a bowl and blend in coconut aminos, garlic, ginger, fish sauce and blend .

2.   Add salmon and let it marinate for 15-20 minutes.

3.   Take a skillet/pan and place it over medium heat.

4.   Add oil and let it heat up.

5.   Add salmon fillets and cook on high heat for 3-4 minutes per side.

6.   Remove dish once crispy.

7.   Add sauce and wine.

8.   Simmer for five minutes on low heat.

9.   Return salmon to the glaze and flip until each side are glazed.

10.   Serve and enjoy!

Nutrition (Per Serving)

Calories: 372

Fat: 24g

Carbohydrates: 3g

Protein: 35g

Generous Stuffed Salmon Avocado

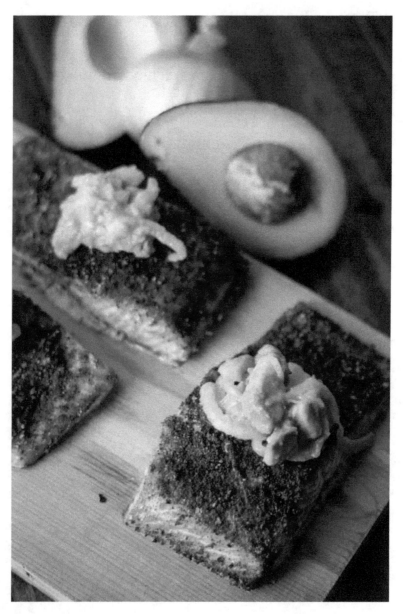

Serving: 2

Prep Time: 10 minutes

Cook Time: 30 minutes

Ingredients:

- ripe organic avocado

- ounces wild caught smoked salmon

- ounce cashew cheese

- tablespoons extra virgin olive oil
- Sunflower seeds as needed

How To:

1.   Cut avocado in half and deseed.

2.   Add the rest of the ingredients to a food processor and process until coarsely chopped.

3.   Place mixture into avocado.

4.   Serve and enjoy!

Nutrition (Per Serving)

Calories: 525

Fat: 48g

Carbohydrates: 4g

Protein: 19g

Spanish Mussels

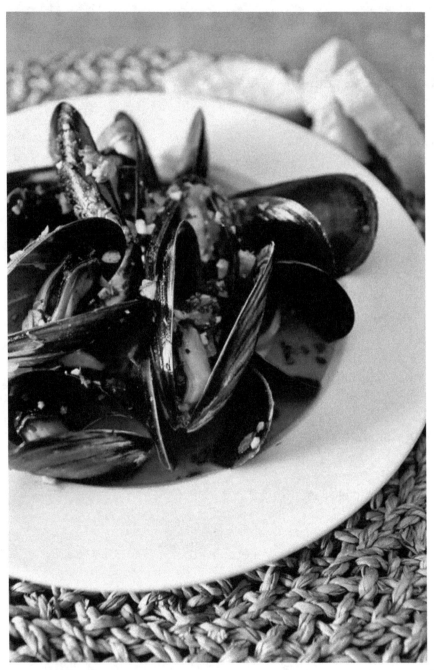

Serving: 4

Prep Time: 10 minutes

Cook Time: 23 minutes

Ingredients:

- tablespoons olive oil

- pounds mussels, scrubbed

- Pepper to taste

- cups canned tomatoes, crushed

- shallot, chopped

- garlic cloves, minced

- cups low sodium vegetable stock

- 1/3 cup cilantro, chopped

How To:

1.   Take a pan and place it over medium-high heat, add shallot and stir-cook for 3 minutes.

2.   Add garlic, stock, tomatoes, pepper, stir and reduce heat, simmer for 10 minutes.

3.   Add mussels, cilantro, and toss.

4.   Cover and cook for 10 minutes more.

5.   Serve and enjoy!

Nutrition (Per Serving)

Calories: 210

Fat: 2g

Carbohydrates: 5g

Protein: 8g

Tilapia Broccoli Platter

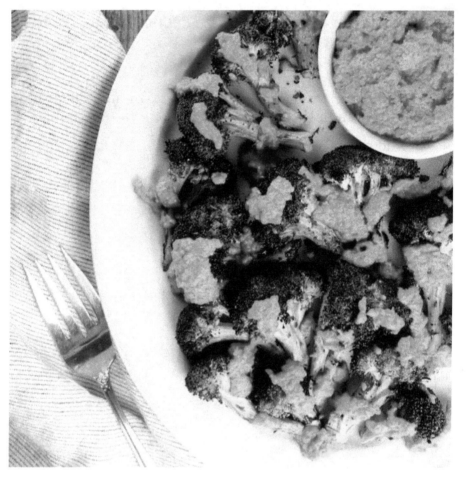

Serving: 2

Prep Time: 4 minutes

Cook Time: 14 minutes

Ingredients:

- Ounce tilapia, frozen

- 1 tablespoon almond butter

- 1 tablespoon garlic, minced

- 1 teaspoon lemon pepper seasoning

- 1 cup broccoli florets, fresh

How To:

1. Pre-heat your oven to 350 degrees F.
2. Add fish in aluminum foil packets.
3. Arrange broccoli around fish.
4. Sprinkle lemon pepper on top.
5. Close the packets and seal.
6. Bake for 14 minutes.
7. Take a bowl and add garlic and almond butter, mix well and keep the mixture on the side.
8. Remove the packet from oven and transfer to platter.

9.   Place almond butter on top of the fish and broccoli, serve and enjoy!

Nutrition (Per Serving)

Calories: 362

Fat: 25g

Carbohydrates: 2g

Protein: 29g

Salmon with Peas and Parsley Dressing

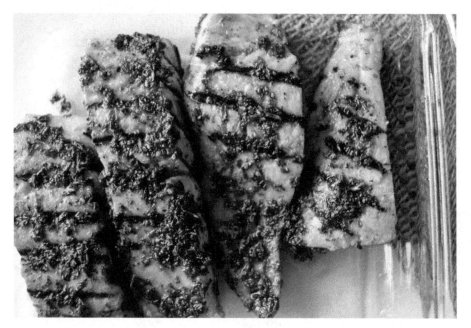

Serving: 4

Prep Time: 15 minutes

Cook Time: 15 minutes

Ingredients:

- 16 ounces salmon fillets, boneless and skin-on

- 1 tablespoon parsley, chopped

- 10 ounces peas

- 9 ounces vegetable stock, low sodium

- 2 cups water

- ½ teaspoon oregano, dried

- ½ teaspoon sweet paprika

- 2 garlic cloves, minced

- A pinch of black pepper

How To:

1.   Add garlic, parsley, paprika, oregano and stock to a kitchen appliance and blend.

2.   Add water to your Instant Pot.

3.   Add steam basket.

4.   Add fish fillets inside the steamer basket.

5.   Season with pepper.

6.   Lock the lid and cook on high for 10 minutes.

7.   Release the pressure naturally over 10 minutes .

8.   Divide the fish amongst plates.

9.   Add peas to the steamer basket and lock the lid again, cook on high for five minutes.

10.   Quick release the pressure.

11.   Divide the peas next to your fillets and serve with the parsley dressing drizzled

12.   on top

13.   Enjoy!

Nutrition (Per Serving)

Calories: 315

Fat: 5g

Carbohydrates: 14g

Protein: 16g

Mackerel and Orange Medley

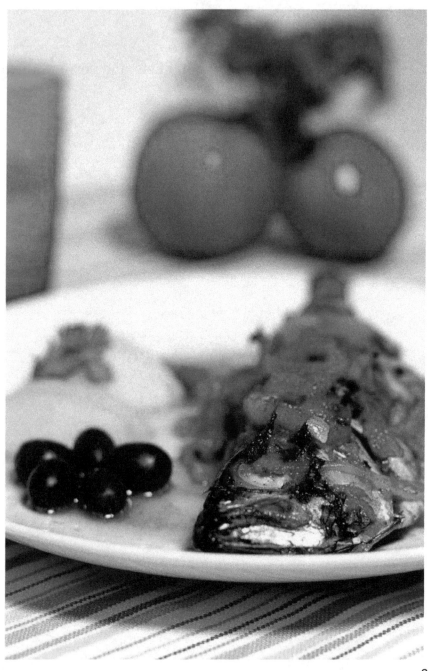

Serving: 4

Prep Time: 10 minutes

Cook Time: 10 minutes

Ingredients:

- mackerel fillets, skinless and boneless

- spring onion, chopped

- 1 teaspoon olive oil

- 1-inch ginger piece, grated

- Black pepper as needed

- Juice and zest of 1 whole orange

- 1 cup low sodium fish stock

How To:

1.   Season the fillets with black pepper and rub vegetable oil .

2.   Add stock, fruit juice , ginger, orange peel and onion to Instant Pot.

3.   Place a steamer basket and add the fillets.

4.   Lock the lid and cook on high for 10 minutes.

5.   Release the pressure naturally over 10 minutes.

6.   Divide the fillets amongst plates and drizzle the orange sauce from the pot over the fish.

7.   Enjoy!

Nutrition (Per Serving)

Calories: 200

Fat: 4g

Carbohydrates: 19g

Protein: 14g

Spicy Chili Salmon

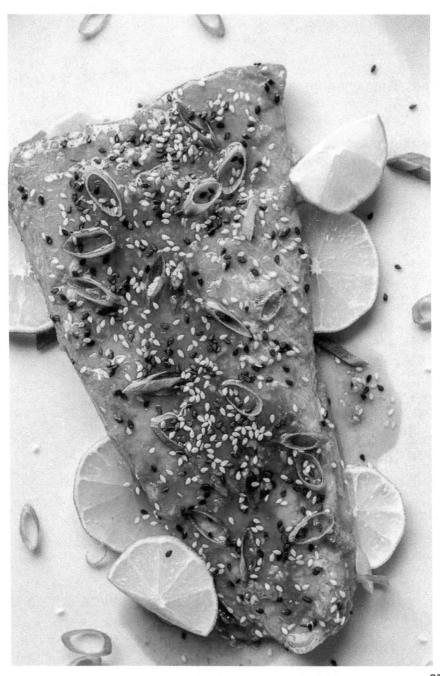

Serving: 4

Prep Time: 10 minutes

Cook Time: 7 minutes

Ingredients:

- salmon fillets, boneless and skin-on

- 2 tablespoons assorted chili peppers, chopped Juice of 1 lemon

- 1 lemon, sliced

- 1 cup water

- Black pepper

How To:

1.   Add water to the moment Pot.

2.   Add steamer basket and add salmon fillets, season the fillets with salt and pepper.

3.   Drizzle juice on top.

4. Top with lemon slices.

5. Lock the lid and cook on high for 7 minutes.

6. Release the pressure naturally over 10 minutes.

7. Divide the salmon and lemon slices between serving plates.

8. Enjoy!

Nutrition (Per Serving)

Calories: 281

Fats: 8g

Carbs: 19g

Protein:7g

Simple One Pot Mussels

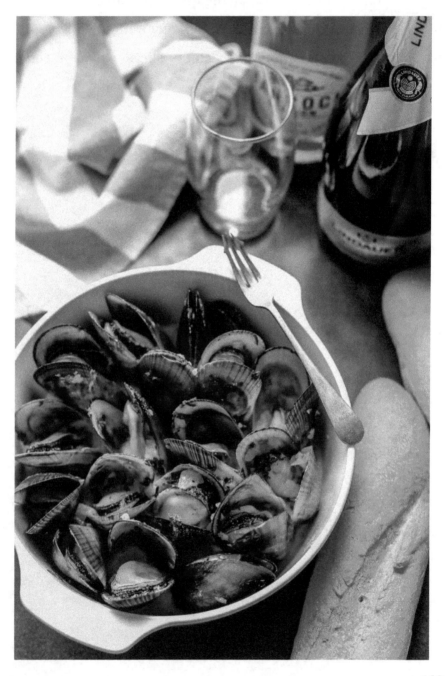

Serving: 4

Prep Time: 10 minutes

Cook Time: 5 minutes

Ingredients:

2 tablespoons butter
2 chopped shallots

minced garlic cloves

½ cup broth

½ cup white wine

2 pounds cleaned mussels

Lemon and parsley for serving

How To:

1.   Clean the mussels and take away the beard.

2.   Discard any mussels that don't close when tapped against a tough surface.

3.   Set your pot to Sauté mode and add chopped onion and butter.

4.   Stir and sauté onions.

5.   Add garlic and cook for 1 minute.

6.   Add broth and wine.

7.   Lock the lid and cook for five minutes on high .

8.   Release the pressure naturally over 10 minutes.

9.   Serve with a sprinkle of parsley and enjoy!

Nutrition (Per Serving)

Calories: 286

Fats: 14g

Carbs: 12g

Protein: 28g

Shrimp With Corn Hash

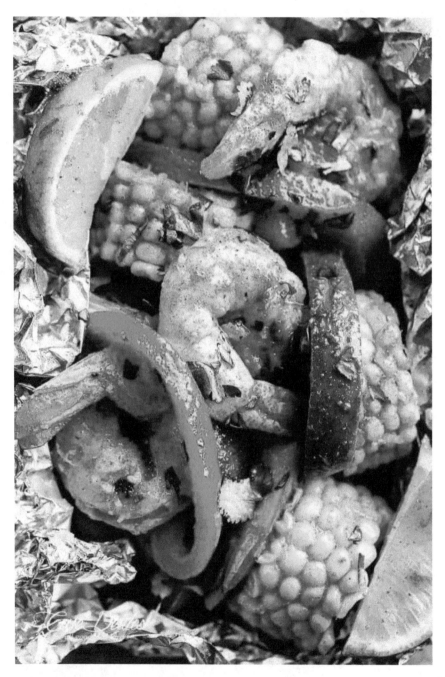

Prep time: 5 minutes

Cook time: 10 minutes

Servings: 4

Ingredients

- Olive oil – 4 tsp.

- Large shrimp - 1 pound, peeled and deveined

- Chopped red onion – ½ cup

- Red bell pepper – ½, chopped

- Fresh corn kernels – 1 ½ cup

- Halved cherry – 1 cup

- Crushed hot red pepper – ¼ tsp.

- Water – ¼ cup Fresh lemon juice – 1 Tbsp.

- Chopped fresh basil – 2 Tbsp.

Method

1. Heat 2 tsp. oil in a skillet.

2. Add the shrimp

3. Cook for 3 to 5 minutes. Transfer to a plate.

4. Heat remaining 2 tsp. oil in the skillet. Add bell pepper.

5. Then onion and stir-fry for 1 minute, or until softened.

6. Add tomatoes, corn, and hot pepper and cover.

7. Cook for 3 minutes.

8. Add the shrimp and reheat, stirring often, about 1 minute.

9. Stir in lemon juice and water and cook.

10. Sprinkle with basil and serve.

Nutritional Facts Per Serving

Calories: 195

Fat: 6g

Carb: 18g

Protein: 18g

Sodium 647mg

Shrimp Ceviche

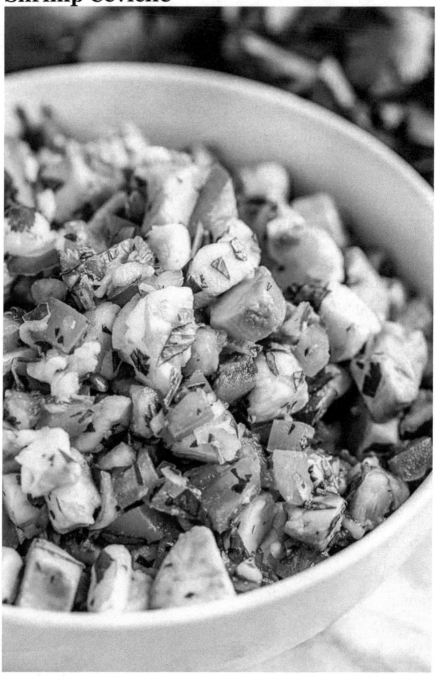

Prep time: 10 minutes

Cook time: 0 minutes

Servings: 8

Ingredients

- Raw shrimp – ½ pound, cut into ¼ inch pieces

- Lemons – 2, zest and juice

- Limes -2, zest and juice

- Olive oil - 2 Tbsp.

- Cumin – 2 tsp.

- Diced red onion – ½ cup

- Diced tomato – 1 cup

- Minced garlic – 2 Tbsp.

- Black beans - 1 cup, cooked

- Diced serrano chili pepper – ¼ cup, seeds removed

- Diced cucumber – 1 cup, peeled and seeded

- Chopped cilantro – ¼ cup

Method

1.   In a bowl, place the shrimp and cover with the lemon and lime juice. Marinate for at least 3 hours.

2.   In another bowl, mix the remaining ingredients and set aside.

3.   Before serving, mix shrimp and the juice with remaining ingredients.

4.   Serve.

Nutritional Facts Per Serving

Calories: 98

Fat: 4g

Carb: 10g

Protein: 7g

Sodium 167mg

CPSIA information can be obtained
at www.ICGtesting.com
Printed in the USA
LVHW081150110521
687091LV00004B/669